BIKE TO LOSE WEIGHT

By

Bruce Fleming

DISCLAIMER

Although the author and publisher have made every effort to ensure that the information in this book was correct at press time, the author and publisher do not assume and hereby disclaim any liability to any party for any loss, damage, or disruption caused by errors or omissions, whether such errors or omissions result from negligence, accident, or any other cause.

This book is not intended as a substitute for the medical advice of physicians. The reader should regularly consult a physician in matters relating to his/her health and particularly with respect to any symptoms that may require diagnosis or medical attention.

The information in this book is meant to supplement, not replace, proper cycling training. Like any sport involving speed, equipment, balance and environmental factors, cycling poses some inherent risk. The author and publisher advise readers to take full responsibility for their safety and know their limits. Before practicing the skills described in this book, be sure that your equipment is well maintained, and do not take risks beyond your level of experience, aptitude, training, and comfort level.

CONTENTS

1. Author's Introduction

"Bike to Lose Weight" is the result of a personal journey that changed my life. I started that journey as a slightly overweight, non-participant observer. Before long I found myself cycling with new friends. I regularly took part in a growing number of events—over distances I'd previously only dreamt of.

In the beginning I struggled to cover 5km on flat ground. Four years later I completed a 12 hour mountain bike ride through the mountains of Nepal. You can read about it my <u>Nepal Mountain Bike</u> post on www.cycletrainingplans.com.

I have many fond memories of that time. It was a period of physical change—I lost 20 kilos in weight, and crucially, kept the weight off. But it was a time of inspirational change too. So inspired was I by the potential for cycling to change lives that I wrote this book to help others on similar journeys.

If you've had trouble losing weight or keeping fit, cycling may just work for you. In the pages that follow I'll explain *why* cycling is such a great activity for losing weight, keeping fit and making new friends.

I'll explain the basics from bike parts to gear. You'll find some simple programs to structure your activity. Eating properly is such an important part of losing weight that I'll show you the ABC's of food and offer some great tips to speed up weight loss. And for those whose cycling may take them beyond the social level, I have included core exercises to encourage body strength and improve your cycling.

For all my tips and guidance, you will still need determination to succeed. Struggling with motivation can be a challenge to anyone embarking on a new activity. So I've included some great motivational tips and exercises to keep you on track. Also, because we cannot predict the weather I have included a section on indoor training so you can you can keep your activity levels high even on bad weather days.

If this all sounds serious, that's because it is. Cycling can change your life. However, cycling can, and should be fun too. For this reason I have asked my good friend Bruiser to come along for the ride. Chapter by chapter he will provide light-hearted interludes as he shares the challenges he faced in following my advice.

Stick with me and by the end of the book you should have the confidence to give biking to lose weight a go. You don't need any special talent to ride a bike and weight loss is not as hard as you think.

Good luck,

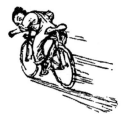

Bruce Fleming.

Bruiser's Introduction

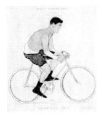

Forty years after I fell off my bike, I climbed back in the saddle again.

Sorry folks, that's not right. Makes it sound like I lay on the street for four decades clutching a grazed knee and moaning like a cow in labour (I'm Bruiser, by the way. Pleased to meet you). What I'm trying to say is that for a long time I just didn't see cycling as a means to get fit and healthy—until I read this book and resolved to use my bike to help me lose weight.

At the time, my bike was a pre-loved Crimson Polecat II. I had rescued her from my friend Barry's garage where she had been lying since the outbreak of World War Two. Polecats were all the rage in Gdansk in the 50s Barry said.

One morning, as I steered the Polecat past a butcher's window on my way to the local velodrome, a thirty-two ounce T-bone steak grabbed my attention using some kind of tractor beam. As I stood rooted to the spot I was startled to see a stranger reflected in the plate glass.

Was that me? No! It couldn't be. The person staring back at me looked like Tweedledum and Tweedledee shoehorned into a single pair of shorts. It was me. It looked as if my Kardashian-sized butt might at any moment crumple the Polecat's frame like an aluminium take-away carton.

This turned out to be a pivotal moment.

I looked frantically about, fearing that some unseen joker with an I-phone was at that very moment uploading smoking-gun evidence of my girth to YouTube. If my aunt Molly called from England to say she'd been shocked to see my butt on the InterWeb and asking when it was, exactly, that I became spherical, I would die of shame. I felt like throwing the Polecat into a ditch and running home to hide under my bed forever.

I stood there, my nose pressed to the butcher's shop window. My Megadeath T-shirt struggling to contain my ever-expanding midriff (I looked like a comic book superhero—Captain Fatso?). I fought back an overwhelming desire to go home to bed with a mug of hot chocolate, a family bag of Doritos and a catering-sized tub of hot fudge.

I had to lose weight. At first I just didn't realise that you could use a bicycle to do it—until I read this book and decided to have a go. It wasn't all plain sailing. Given my appalling lack of will power I expected to start badly and fade away—that's the norm for me. Nor was I prepared for the discovery that the double-dealing, side-winding, devious part of my subconscious (which I named Chuffer for ease of reference) was steadfastly at work trying to undermine my efforts because he liked me being a couch potato. In the chapters that follow, you'll learn more about how I eventually lost weight and got fit but for now, oil that chain and get ready for the ride of your life. Let's see what this book's about.

2. Why cycling is ideal for losing weight

Riding a bike is a great way to lose weight. Here's some reasons why:

- Most people can ride a bike. We learn as children. Once learned, never forgotten.
- Even if you have never ridden a bike, you can quickly learn.
- It's a non-impact sport. The body doesn't suffer the impact stress of other activities such as jogging, making it ideal for people with weight or joint problems.

Cycling burns fat

Cyclists use the big muscle groups in their legs, hips and core. This causes muscles and the networks of blood vessels that feed them, to grow. Prolonged activity as in a steady ride causes these muscles to burn fat for energy.

As well as weight loss, high blood pressure is more easily controlled, cardiac and lung function improves.

Cycling is a great activity to lose weight. The activity burns calories resulting in weight loss. It's a great activity that you're more likely to continue on a regular basis. Reduced stress, better sleep and improved general health are all common benefits from cycling regularly.

The muscles continue to burn fat for up to 24 hours after you stop cycling. As you get fitter, the body increases its capability to process more oxygen and this increases the amount of calories burnt. Lean muscle mass, which is more efficient at burning calories, increases.

High-intensity cycling is unnecessary for burning fat. In fact a longer ride at a steady pace burns fat more effectively than high-intensity riding.

You may also be pleased to learn that fat disappears from your belly first!

Appetite decrease

It's a common misconception that cycling demands a larger food intake. In fact, studies show that cycling can *suppress* the appetite for a few hours after the activity. At the same time, an increase in pleasure hormones makes you feel good. The combination of these factors ensures that you are less likely to binge on snack foods for an emotional boost.

Stress reduction

Regular cycling helps reduce stress. The physical exertion uses up excess adrenaline and slows cortisol (the stress hormone) production. This decrease in stress will help you get a better night's sleep.

Studies show that lack of sleep triggers weight gain. Fatigue stimulates the body to produce a hormone which causes hunger. So you eat more and put on weight. A bicycle ride of about 30 minutes a day, four days a week over a period of several months has been shown to result in one extra hour of sleep a night. That's seven hours each week— a huge boost to your wellbeing and a healthy contribution to your continued weight loss.

Fun

I mentioned this in the introduction, but it's important enough to mention again: Cycling is fun. Once you become familiar with your bike and get into a cycling routine, enjoyment levels increase. Every ride can take you to new and interesting places ripe for exploration.

This is one of the great benefits of bike riding. Many exercise programs have more than their fair share of boredom. Not so with cycling. Weight loss becomes a *byproduct* of cycling and before you know it, you'll find yourself enjoying the pursuit and regulating your weight in the process.

New friends.

As you cycle more often, you will make contact with other riders, with other circles of friends with whom you can share your experiences. Coffee rides are a great way to meet new friends. Your new found acquaintances will be happy to offer advice. I found many good friends amongst people I met on cycling rides.

If you are new to an area, the local bike shop is a great place to learn about cycling groups. These groups often arrange trips to places you'd never dream of.

Excuses

You're probably dreaming up reasons why waiting until tomorrow before you start cycling is a good idea—of turning this into your personal Mañana Project. Don't worry. This is more common than you think. Here's a few of the excuses I hear from people to justify not cycling.

- "I can't ride a bike."
- "I don't know how to change gears."
- "I don't know when to change gears."
- "I'm worried about the cleats and pedals."
- "What if I fall off?"
- "I can't ride up hills."
- "I don't want to look like an idiot in Lycra."
- "I'm too old to start cycling."

Most people can ride a bike. If they can't they can soon learn. If you're inexperienced, start on an open flat grassed area with a gentle slope. Practice coasting down the slope, not with your feet on the pedals, but using your legs for balance. Once you become comfortable with this, repeat the exercise with your feet on the pedals. You can progress to pedaling along a flat stretch.

Once confident riding a flat stretch, start learning about the gears. Using a bike set up on stationery rollers is a good method of learning gear changes without worrying about falling off the bike. Get used to riding along the flat and changing gears before progressing to hills. Before you know it cycling will become second nature to you.

Not being able to disengage your cleats from the pedals is a common misgiving. If you are concerned, start off cycling with standard pedals until you become accustomed to riding with cleats. It's a good idea to use a stationary bike with cleats or get someone to hold your bike steady while you practice engaging and disengaging them.

Accidents

Few things in life come risk free and cycling is no exception. Most cyclists fall off at some stage but that's no reason not to cycle. If you thought about the alarming number of car accidents before you climbed into a car, you'd probably never drive.

Remember that the more you ride the more confident your cycling will become. Start off in areas where there is little or no traffic until your confidence grows. Many people prefer riding mountain bike trails so they don't have to contend with vehicles on the road. Riding up hills becomes easier the fitter you become. Start off riding flat routes and progress to hills as you feel more confident.

Age is no barrier to cycling. There are many people who are active riders well into their 80s and you'd not have to search far to find a ninety year old cyclist. As for the Lycra excuse, you don't have to wear Lycra—you can wear whatever feels comfortable. However you will find clothing designed for cycling such as Lycra gives you comfort and a more enjoyable ride than street gear with less chance of chafing. Once you become a regular cyclist you will be proud to be seen in Lycra.

I have some motivational tips for you next but first you might like to hear Bruiser's take on motivation. Maybe you can relate to his journey to fitness.

3. Motivation

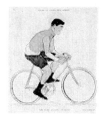

Motivation. That's what I needed—something that would get man and Polecat to trek the thirty yards between my couch and the road without a stopover at the fridge to make a sandwich for the journey. I must admit that somewhere near the end of my thirties my get-up-and-go got up and went and despite fingertip searches across three counties it hasn't been seen since.

So I treated this section of the book with its useful tips on how to get and stay motivated, with respect. There were times when I wished the Polecat, like a machine from Transformers: Dark of the Moon, would metamorphose into a completely different contraption before my very eyes—a Lazy Boy recliner perhaps, or a massage chair. But I stuck with it.

I entered a competition as the author suggested. So I'd stay focused. Unfortunately, Chuffer got involved and I ended up applying for a one mile mini-marathon in the spring of 2025. Chuffer was cool with this because I couldn't really start training any time soon or I'd reach peak fitness a decade too early. Thanks a bunch Chuffer.

Chuffer struck again after I agreed with my next door neighbour, Barry, to a strict regimen of weekly twenty mile rides over hilly terrain. As the agreed date loomed, I bottled it, turning the lights out and hiding behind the sofa five minutes before Barry wheeled his bike up to my front door (What? Barry didn't turn up to my barbecue last month despite sending him an invitation three weeks in advance, so he has nothing to complain about.)

This section was packed tighter than a goose feather pillow with words of inspiration. Most stirring. Some scary—Like Stephen R.Covey's "Motivation is a fire from within. If someone else tries to light that fire under you, chances are it will burn very briefly."

What was Covey on about? Was this about an arsonist, spontaneous combustion, or both? Whichever, his quote did nothing to set my heart racing.

By contrast, another quote seemed to nail the whole point of exercise: "Too many people confine their exercise to jumping to conclusions, running up bills, stretching the truth, bending over backwards, lying down on the job, sidestepping responsibility and pushing their luck." Now that's the kind of exercise regime I'm talking about.

Ok let's get serious now and read how motivation can help us with getting in shape.

We need motivation to get us off the couch and into the saddle—a difficult process if you're new to cycling, especially if losing weight is your main motivation. Sometimes leaping into your Lycra before leaping on your bike comes below poking yourself in the eye with a stick on your list of smart things to do today. And it's worse if you don't feel comfortable on the bike.

Here are a few pointers to boost your motivation.

Write down a Goal

Write down a goal and associate it with weight loss, bike riding or both. Common goals include riding a distance or losing a certain amount of weight. By writing them down and pinning them on the wall where you can see them, you are setting yourself up to succeed.

Choose an Event to Participate in

By choosing an event you make a commitment that helps you to stay motivated. It doesn't matter whether it's a competitive or a social ride. Cycling events and fun rides are constantly being organized, so check with your local bike shop for a list of events.

Organize your Time

People often complain that they can't find time to ride for a few hours. This is undoubtedly true. But a high activity thirty minute session can often prove more beneficial than an hour or two of aimless riding.

The key here is to make the most of the time you have available. If you have only thirty minutes to spare, spend five minutes warming up, then do six or eight hard bursts for 30 seconds with 90 seconds at an easy pace in between. This produces a great fitness boost and you won't feel guilty at missing a ride.

If the day slips by without meeting your daily goal, you can always do a session on the spin bike or indoor trainer.

Arrange a regular ride with Friends.

Organizing a regular day or time to cycle with friends increases the chances of you turning up for the ride.

Make your ride a Habit

Choose a favourite ride and turn it into a habit. Use this as a base for developing your commitment to riding. Although riding the same course at the same intensity won't get you fitter, your commitment to regular riding will set you up to achieve your goals.

Once you're familiar with a course, time yourself over

sections. Choose a hill or flat section and aim to beat your section time each ride. This provides you with smaller targets within your ride and these too will help you stay motivated.

Share your plans with friends and family.

You'll be more likely to succeed if you know others have an interest in your progress. Telling your friends and family about events you intend to participate in will encourage you to stick with your plan. You might provide the motivation for someone else to get involved.

Motivational Quotes

Motivational quotes offer a great source of inspiration when facing any sort of challenge. Here are some of my favourite motivational quotes I hope will inspire you. Find one that resonates with you, write it out and pin it somewhere you can regularly see it.

> *"People often say that motivation doesn't last. Well, neither does bathing—that's why we recommend it daily." (Zig Ziglar)*

> *"Motivation is a fire from within. If someone else tries to light that fire under you, chances are it will burn very briefly." (Stephen R. Covey)*

> *"Motivation is like food for the brain. You cannot get enough in one sitting. It needs continual and regular top up's." (Peter Davies)*

> *"Motivation is what gets you started. Habit is what keeps you going." (Jim Rohn)*

> *"In order to change we must be sick and tired of being sick and tired." (Unknown)*

Exercise & motivation

While we're looking at quotations let's start this new section with another:

> "Those who think they have not time for bodily exercise will sooner or later have to find time for illness." (Edward Stanley)

> "Too many people confine their exercise to jumping to conclusions, running up bills, stretching the truth, bending over backwards, lying down on the job, sidestepping responsibility and pushing their luck." (Anonymous)

> "Fitness—If it came in a bottle, everybody would have a great body." (Cher)

Motivational Challenges

> "Stumbling is not falling." (Portuguese Proverb)

> "As long as a man stands in his own way, everything seems to be in his way." (Ralph Waldo Emerson)

> "If you find a path with no obstacles, it probably doesn't lead anywhere." (Unknown)

> "The significant problems we face cannot be solved by the same level of thinking that created them." (Albert Einstein)

> "Whatever course you decide upon, there is always someone to tell you that you are wrong. There are always difficulties arising which tempt you to believe that your critics are right. To map out a course of action and follow it to an end requires courage." (Ralph Waldo Emerson)

> "Don't dwell on what went wrong. Instead, focus on what to do next. Spend your energies on moving forward toward finding the answer." (Denis Waitley)

"Stand up to your obstacles and do something about them. You will find that they haven't half the strength you think they have." (Norman Vincent Peale)

"The older you get, the tougher it is to lose weight because by then, your body and your fat are really good friends." (Anonymous)

"What you eat in private will show up in public." (Unknown)

"Don't wait until everything is just right. It will never be perfect. There will always be challenges, obstacles and less than perfect conditions. So what. Get started now. With each step you take, you will grow stronger and stronger, more and more skilled, more and more self-confident and more and more successful." (Mark Victor Hansen)

"Only those who risk going too far can possibly find out how far one can go..." (T.S. Eliot)

"That which we persist in doing becomes easier to do; not that the nature of the thing itself is changed, but that our power to do is increased." (Ralph Waldo Emerson)

"Focus on where you want to go, not on what you fear." (Anthony Robbins)

Affirmations.

Don't underestimate the power of affirmations to help change your life. An affirmation is a short positive phrase you repeat to yourself. When you first start making positive affirmations, they may not yet be true. But with repetition, affirmations are stored in your subconscious mind, and you start to believe them. Eventually they become your reality.

Over time, affirmations overwrite self-defeating and negative self-beliefs. They replace negative thoughts with positive thoughts and beliefs which provide confidence, belief, positivity and ambition.

Examples

"Every day, in every way, I'm getting better and better" (Emile Coue)

"I am a great cyclist"

"I love cycling and it helps me reach my ideal weight"

"I easily control my weight with healthy eating and exercising"

Make up an affirmation of your own. Repeat it first thing in the morning, last thing at night and during the day. Overall, aim to repeat your affirmation ten times each day. Write it on a sheet of paper and pin it to your wall.

If you're intent on becoming a good cyclist with a toned physique, you'll need to change who you are. And you change who you are by changing the way you think and act. One technique for doing that is to act as if you are already that person.

Act as if you're slim, long enough, and one day you may become slim even though you may be overweight today. Similarly, if you act as if you're a great cyclist long enough, then one day you will become a great cyclist. To quote Bob Proctor, "Act like the person you want to become".

Here's a great technique. You'll need two photographs. One of a cyclist or person with a physique you would like to have. The other should be a photograph of yourself from which you cut your head and superimpose it on the first photograph. If possible, use a photo editor and print out a realistic picture.

Pin this image where you can see it every day. Your subconscious mind will take this image of yourself on board and influence your actions to become the person in the photograph.

In the next chapter I'll explain the variety of bikes available and what gear you need for cycling. My friend Bruiser has a few smart remarks to make on the subject first.

4. BIKES and GEAR.

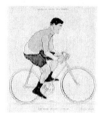

I have to say, even before reaching this section, I was beginning to see the Crimson Polecat II in a different light. I often spent time staring at her as I explained earlier but I could now see why the kindest thing would be to dump her in a skip. Sometimes you've just got to move on.

Let's face it, she wasn't a pretty sight. The chain hung limply over the cogs like a dead snake. The seat was comparable in size to a bar-stool. The handlebars had been styled on cow horns. There were ten spokes on the front wheel and twelve on the rear. It had no gears and when ridden, pulled you into the side of the road like a surly farm-horse.

But what would I replace her with? I had a hankering for something between a Bone-shaker and one of those modern hi-tech marvels. You know the sort of contraption—like something out of Terminator, weighing less than a handful of feathers and, powered by the right legs, capable of 80 mph.

I understood that several types of bike were available. I could opt for a road bike—what other kind could there be? Or possibly a mountain bike. Logically, if a road bike is for the road, then a mountain bike must be the mountains. Duh!

I immediately struck mountain bikes off wish list. In my condition I wasn't planning to cycle the entire length of the Andean mountain chain any time soon. I decided on a road bike. I wasn't going to buy one just yet; I didn't have the money, but that's what I would buy when my home finances recovered. For the time being, the Crimson Polecat and I were *to remain a team.*

Choosing a bike is just the beginning, of course. I should get a bike mechanic to check it over too, the author insisted. Who else was I going to get to do this if not a bike mechanic—a florist?

Actually, when I read a second suggestion that I should also ask the bike mechanic to adjust the bike to suit my body it struck me that it might take somebody with the creativity of a florist to complete this Herculean task—I weigh 210 pounds and not a single pound hangs the right way.

Then there's headgear and shorts to take in to account. I was exhausted just thinking of all the stuff I needed to do and I hadn't turned a wheel yet. I was already uneasy about my current helmet—a WWI German Army job with a spike like a lightning conductor up top. It would have to go, if only to avoid embarrassment. My cycling shorts were less of an embarrassment but they were essentially beach shorts. Fine for stretching your legs along the promenade in May. But as abrasive on the inner thighs as a pot scrubber when cycling.

My nickname—Bruiser—conjures up in some people, the image of a heavyweight boxer. In fact, the name arose because of my childhood habit of falling off my bike ("In the black and blue corner, 'The Bruiser!'"). I'm far more emotionally sensitive than my nickname suggests. And never was that sensitivity better demonstrated, than when I recently bought my first Lycra cycling outfit.

In the pioneering days of recreational cycling, an enthusiast might wear more clothing than a nineteenth century Tyrollean mountain climber. If you had a shape back then, that was your business; the casual observer couldn't tell what it was through all that corduroy, leather and wool. Unfortunately, for those of us cycling to fitness in the modern era, masking our body shape is impossible. This is in great part due to the perils of Lycra ('The Perils of Lycra!' Sounds like one of the labours of Hercules, doesn't it?)

Lycra is the world's most unforgiving fabric, merciless in its capacity to expose the 'real you'. Nothing will more cruelly draw attention to your wobbly bits than Lycra. Great if you're Nicole Scherzinger. Not so great if you're a middle-aged sheep farmer with a roll of midriff fat like the inner tube of a monster truck.

The cost of cycling my way back to fitness was escalating, but I was determined. So I resolved to recover my cheque book from under the floorboards in the shed, blow off the cobwebs and start spending money on a good cause—getting the right tools for the job.

You better have a look at the next section on gear so at least you know the basics.

BIKES

Choose a bike suitable for your preferred type of riding. Any bike will get you from A to B but you might as well get one that is comfortable and suited to your ride.

Road Bikes.

Designed to be ridden on the road, these light, easy-to-manoeuvre, aerodynamic and responsive bikes make for a fast, efficient ride.

Mountain Bikes.

Designed to be ridden off road. Their design reflects the rougher terrain they have to handle: Shock absorbers and large tires to smooth a rough ride; flatter handlebars and frame design to position the rider in a more upright position compared to a road bike.

You can ride these on the road but they will give you a slower ride. If you plan to do on- road and off-road riding, consider a hybrid bike.

Hybrid Bikes.

A cross between mountain bikes and road bikes. They don't have the suspension features of a full mountain bike but they will enable you to ride at a reasonable pace on the road while providing a comfortable off-road ride. They have flatter handle bars and medium width tires for a more upright ride. Hybrid bikes are more suitable for new riders as the riding position is more upright and instills more confidence in the inexperienced.

Bike check.

If you're purchasing a second hand bike, get a competent bike mechanic or regular cyclist to check it out. Over time, cables rust and bearings seize. By getting your bike checked thoroughly before use you'll lessen the chance of gear failure spoiling your ride and denting your confidence.

Make sure that the bike has been adjusted to suit your body. In striving for easy foot contact with the ground when coming off the pedals, new riders often set their seats too low. Correct seat and handlebar positions are essential to ensure a comfortable ride that won't put strain on your body parts.

Clothing & Gear

Choose clothing and gear that is comfortable and that will keep you safe. Consider the terrain you'll be cycling through and what the climate is like there. Check the weather before you leave and take appropriate clothing. Here are some items to make your ride more pleasurable.

Helmet

Road surfaces can be unforgiving. Most riders come off their bike sooner or later and a good helmet helps prevent serious head injuries. Make sure the straps are tight enough to prevent the helmet sliding back on your head.

Socks

While you could use any socks, sports socks are better in the long run.

Gloves

Fingerless work best. But if it's cold, use full finger gloves (thermal if possible).

Cycling jersey

Cycling jerseys are longer in the back so they don't ride up your back and expose your skin to the elements when you lean forward. They have pockets in the lower back and sides for easy access.

Jacket

A lightweight jacket is essential to protect you from the rain. The best of these are of an ultra-lightweight type that can be folded into your back pocket. Make sure when buying any product designed to keep you dry, that you know the difference between 'waterproof' and 'water resistant'.

To be considered waterproof an item must be made of waterproof fabric with sealed seams. 'Water resistant' items are made from materials that *repel* water but which are not waterproof.

Cycle shoes.

New cyclists are often concerned about clipless cycling shoes.

What if they are unable to disengage in time before dismounting? If you are concerned you could start with cage pedals, though most riders progress to clipless due to the greater efficiency and comfort they provide.

Tools and spares

Most cyclists carry a few tools and spares. These are kept in a small bag that hooks under the bicycle seat. Bare essentials include:

- Spare tube
- CO_2 tire inflator if you don't have a pump attached to the bike frame
- Two tire levers
- Small multi-tool
- Water bottle and cage (attached to the bike frame)

Shorts

Cycling shorts use chamois leather as protection against chafing and to offer a more comfortable ride. Lycra prevents abrasion on the skin and prevents moisture being held close to the skin. Trust me—once accustomed to cycling in these shorts you will never go back to regular shorts.

Visit your local cycle shop and check out the different types of bikes available. Get the expert to show you the difference. While you're there have a look at the gear available and ask what's suitable for your level of riding.

The next chapter is an A to Z of bikes parts so you know what to refer to and don't end up sounding like Bruiser does in the following piece.

5. KNOW THE PARTS OF A BIKE.

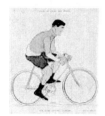

In the same way that a junior doctor must learn to name all the bones of the human skeleton, a cyclist should be able to name all the parts of his bike. If only to make sure he can order spare parts without embarrassment. Don't let ignorance lead to conversations like this.

'Mr. Shopkeeper, can I have one of those doo-dads that's a bit like an oxygen cylinder only slimmer? They're used to force air into tyres. They're kind of like … well, a … bicycle pump?'

'You mean a bicycle pump?'

'Yes, that's it! Could I have one of those please?

I like the way this section explains all the parts of a bicycle and I amazed myself by knowing some of them already—like 'wheels' and 'handlebars'. I didn't count all the parts but it looked from the diagram like there might be a couple of thousand. Chuffer was keen to avoid learning the names, suggesting instead that I take the diagram to the repair shop and point at the parts I wanted with one of those things that looks like an oxygen cylinder, only slimmer.

And by the way, no way am I going to try to pronounce 'derailleur' in a crowded shop. Sounds like a hero of the French Revolution.

Just one niggle. I am concerned about the 'crank from the wrong side of town' referred to in this section. I hope they get him. I won't be cycling after dark until they do. After all, I don't want my bicycle clips stolen.

Let's see what Bruce has to say about Bicycle parts.

Bicycle Parts

So, we've reached the stage when you just want to mount that bike and ride your heart out. There's just one problem—you haven't a clue how to tell one part of a bike from another. You think a derailleur is someone who's gone off the rails. Have faith. It's not that difficult. You will quickly learn to identify each part and how it functions. The photo below identifies all the main parts.

- **Handlebars:** These come in a variety of shapes but the function is the same. They are what you hold onto to steer and control the bike.

- **Levers or shifters:** Levers or shifters come attached to handlebars. Their function is to change the gears. Usually the left lever moves the chain from the big chain ring in the front to the smaller one for big gear shifts. The right lever controls the chain shift on the back cogs which is used for smaller gear shifts.

- **Brake Levers:** Used to slow the bike in combination with the gear shifter. The left one usually works the rear brake and the right one, the front.

- **Brake:** These pads slow the wheel. With hydraulic brakes the brake disc is located on the central part of the wheel.

- **Derailleur**: These guide the chain to each of the chain rings in the front and cogs on the back cassette.

- **Cassette**: The cogs on the back wheel.

- **Chain ring:** The big rings attached to the pedal. The biggest ring is the hardest to pedal.

- **Seat or Saddle:** This is what you sit on. They come in all shapes and sizes. Pick one that suits you.

- **Cranks and Pedals:** The pedal is the flat section you place your foot. The crank is the arm the pedal is attached to. Some pedals are designed for clip-in shoes while others are clip-less, attaching to a special cleat on riding shoes.

- **Wheels**: The outer section holds the tyres and is connected to the central hub by the spokes.

- **Tyres**: These are the outer parts of the wheel that make ground contact and contain the inflated tube inside. They vary in size and shape depending on the type of bike and riding surface.

- **Forks**: These are the part of the bike the wheel is attached to.

- **Tubes**: The frame of the bike

- **Cables**: These are the wires that connect the levers to the brakes and derailleurs

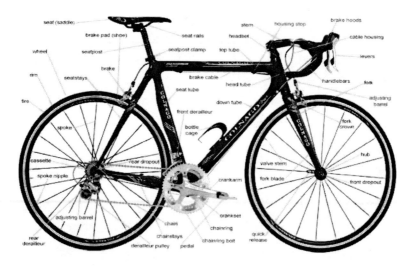

Take this diagram, get your bike out of the garage and start to identify the parts so you become familiar with them. If you learn the main parts you won't be embarrassed.

In the next chapter I'll give you some basics about food and how to change the way you eat to help you lose weight. Firstly

Bruiser has his take on eating for weight loss.

6. WHAT TO EAT TO LOSE WEIGHT.

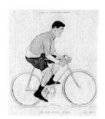

There's a bunch of food facts in this chapter. Lots of interesting recipes for healthy eating. I always knew I was a salad dodger but before I decided to follow the author's wisdom, I wasn't sure how much of a salad dodger I really was (though the butcher's window affair made me wonder) until I found a quiz on the Interweb. There were three questions:

    a.*Would Ripley's Believe It Or Not? pay handsomely for a photograph of your thunderous thighs so they could upload it next to photos of the hang-gliding raccoon and the woman who ate a tree?*

    b.*Does it worry you that one more litre of Pumpkin Cheesecake ice cream might tip you into having your own gravitational field?*

    c.*Does your face turn scarlet when you try to blow out a single candle?*

I answered 'yes' to all three. The results table classified me as a citizen of Lard City. This was unsurprising. According to the graph on my doctor's wall which plotted weight against health risk, my chances of badness happening were three miles north of huge.

When I read this chapter I realized I was guilty of rewarding myself for effort by eating just like the author said. For instance I'd cycle round the block then convince myself I'd earned a double cheeseburger with maxi-fries and a jumbo milkshake. When I calculated the calories I realized that I would have had to cycle up Kilimanjaro to burn that many calories.

I had to read the section twice but I got the point in the end—there are thousands of weight loss products to choose from but there are only a few simple rules for mastering healthy eating:

- *Eat fresh fruit and vegetables (I seemed to remember seeing an orange once in a documentary. So I made a mental note here to do better).*
- *Watch your sugar consumption*
- *Eat fresh chicken or fish*
- *Eat small amounts of nuts and seeds daily (Somehow, sucking on a couple of sunflower seeds for lunch as a substitute for a jumbo sausage filled me with dread).*

I've given you a heads up of what's in the next section but have a read so you know for sure what you're meant to be eating.

Eating and Weight Loss.

You want to lose weight. That's why you've decided to try bike riding. But the way ahead isn't clear—everywhere you look you find another diet. Which to choose? Many of these diets work. Participants lose weight. Though more often than not fluid alone is lost and rapidly replaced whenever the diet stops.

Most diets fail because they don't address the causes of weight gain. Nor are they sustainable beyond the short term.

Bike Riding: A means to lose weight

Bike riding *helps* with weight loss. I love this method because it has so many benefits once regular patterns of activity are laid down. Once routines are established, those excess kilos will melt away.

You must remain vigilant about your eating habits, however. The moment you believe that your increased activity levels entitle you to eat unsuitable food, you run the risk of sabotaging all your good work.

Food Facts

Understanding some basic facts about food will help you maintain a suitable weight.

The main foods groups are carbohydrates, protein, fats and oils.

Carbohydrates

The carbohydrate food group causes most confusion when it comes to weight loss. Many of us are taught that our diet should consist mainly of carbohydrate, with some protein and a little fat or oil.

However, not all carbohydrates are the same. Some, like white bread and pasta, lack fibre. These are rapidly converted to sugar by the body. If this sugar is not immediately required for energy it is stored as fat.

Vegetables contain complex carbohydrates which also contain fibre and other nutrients such as minerals and vitamins. These take longer for the body to digest so there is no rapid rise in blood sugar levels and less opportunity to binge on snacks in compensation for the sudden drop in blood sugar that takes place after eating simple carbohydrates such as white bread.

Bread made from wheat is a staple for many people. Unfortunately it doesn't help with keeping weight down. Many athletes find they have far more energy and have leaner bodies when they restrict or eliminate wheat products from their diet.

Protein

Proteins are formed from amino acids—the building blocks of the body. These are required to repair and replace tissue. Most people grossly overestimate the amount of protein they need. Meat, fish, chicken, nuts and seeds are the most popular sources of protein. The daily requirements of the average person could fit into a portion the size of a clenched fist.

Fats

The benefits or otherwise of a diet rich in fats and oils has recently become a controversial topic. For years we were told to avoid fat, eat margarine and generally follow a low fat diet. Now, the conventional wisdom is that we should be consuming a reasonable amount of 'good' fats such as pure grass-fed cow's butter, pure coconut oil, olive oil and avocado.

These saturated fats, once considered unhealthy, are making a comeback.

Having said that, you should continue to avoid unhealthy fats, especially hydrogenated vegetable oils and margarine. Unfortunately the healthy eater is not helped by the fact that the processed food industry is a huge consumer of unhealthy trans-fats. Many convenience foods contain trans-fats.

The problem is that the body finds trans-fats hard to metabolize. They interfere with a process known as thermogenesis in which fat stored in the body is broken down when required for energy. In practice you experience the body's demands for more energy as a sugar craving which forces you to eat carbohydrates to satisfy that demand.

In turn this process results in insulin resistance. Excess carbohydrate intake results in the storage of excess fat and the amount of insulin available in the body is insufficient to cope with the continued oversupply of sugar from carbohydrates.

What to do.

This all sounds a bit daunting. But there are several things you can do.

- Eat mainly fresh fruit and vegetables
- Don't overeat sweet fruits as these are high in fructose—a type of sugar
- Consume fresh meat, chicken, fish, nuts and seeds daily, **in small quantities**
- Use pure, unsalted butter, virgin coconut oil or olive oil daily. Avoid cooking with olive oil as it has a low smoke point. It will burn at a low temperature. Instead, add it to meals at the end of the cooking. It will taste better and is healthier for you.
- Make sure butter or coconut oil is pure (some are

blended with a vegetable oils such as canola or margarine).

- In short eat *fresh* food. Better still, grow it yourself. Remember, most packaged foods are energy dense and don't contribute to good health.
- Drink plenty of pure water

Maybe you're not sure where to start with your diet. If so, at the end of each day, write down what you've eaten. Be honest with yourself. Nobody else has to see it. At the end of the week review your notes and see if you can identify poor choices. This could be cakes, added sugar and soft drinks for example.

Pick out one area to focus on. For instance, let's say if you realize that you're taking three teaspoons of sugar with your coffee three times a day. Make it your goal to cut your sugar intake to one or two teaspoons. If you've eating a muffin every morning with your coffee try replacing it with a piece of fruit. Concentrate on one or two areas to start with then move on to something else. This will be easier than trying to change everything that's wrong at the same time.

In the next chapter I give a few tips on overcoming sweet cravings which should make it easier to cut out sugar. Bruiser managed to do it (eventually), as he points out next and so can you.

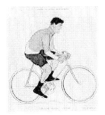

"Sugar, sugar, honey, honey. You are my candy girl". Do you remember that song by the 'Archies"? Probably before your time, but I used to sing it all the time while I lost count of the amount of sugar I shovelled into my coffee at the time. When I

first read this section I could picture myself consuming oily sardines to excise my sugar craving. Yuck!

"Slow down" Bruce says but if I went any slower my shadow would overtake me. I got his point, I was my own worst enemy. I could see there was more to my rampant craving for sugar than met the eye. But wait, there's more. Read on as Bruce explains how you can get that sweet tooth under control.

7. Sugar, Sugar.

What happens if you crave sugar as I'm sure many of you do? You know this is sabotaging your effort to get your weight sorted out but find it really hard to stop the craving. Here are a few tips to help stop the sugar cravings.

1.Eat food that will fuel you for longer

Try adding more fat to your diet. People have been scared to add fats to their diet because of the belief that, eating fat makes you fat. Try adding good fats such as avocado, pure butter, nuts, coconut oil and oily fish especially at lunchtime. This will cause your mid-afternoon sugar craving to decrease. These types of fats slow the release of glucose into your bloodstream causing you to feel satisfied for longer.

2.Slow yourself down.

Over activity causes your body to burn glucose. If you live your life in the fast lane, push your body intensely during cardio exercises, stress out at work or home or even overindulge in caffeine and stimulants it will cause your body to demand glucose.

You need to slow down. This will cause the body to relax and help the body activate the para-sympathetic nervous system which controls the repair and rest of the body.

Controlled breathing and meditation exercises can help you achieve a calmer state of mind. This will help your body to burn fat instead of sugar for fuel meaning you will be less likely to experience those hunger pangs and reach for a sweet snack.

3.What emotion triggers your craving?

Emotional needs that aren't being met are often triggers for sugar craving. We are often conditioned in life to need something sweet to feel happy or satisfied. This often harks back to childhood when sweets are often given as a treat or reward.

When you have an intense desire for sugar, stop and think what may be triggering it. Are you unhappy, depressed, bored or tired?

Identify some non-food related activities that give you a happy feeling and try to include more of these in your life. A trip to the movies, playing with your children or having a holiday to look forward to may be all it needs to get your mind in a better space and diminish you sugar cravings.

Before you go onto the next section try and identify any emotional triggers you may have that cause you to reach for the sweets. Were you angry, bored or depressed? Next time you're in that emotional state find another activity to take your mind off eating.

The Cave Man diet or Paleo is next up. It's worth reading about, it even made an impression on Bruiser as you'll see.

8. HOW THE CAVE MAN DIET CAN HELP.

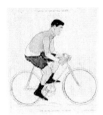

Boy, did this section wake me up. I am beginning to believe there may be life beyond the double cheeseburger after all! The day after I read it, I gave Burger King a wide berth, staying home to make myself something tasty from the recipe list.

As I understand it, the Paleo-Diet is based on the luncheon choices of our Neanderthal hunter-gatherer forebears (not to be confused with the three bears—who belong in the Goldilocks story) who roamed the savannah in search of nuts and berries for 2.5 million years, stealing people's washing and trampling through their flower beds in the process.

I tried the Paleo-diet. I hung around the local park, foraging for berries in the bushes. When this began to draw attention from various municipal authorities I gave up.

You can't have milk on this diet because they didn't take milk back then. You'd think they'd have got fed up with peanuts after all that time—remember they were unsalted back then too. Those who know what they are talking about (not me, obviously) say that the Paleo-Diet perfectly matches our evolved digestive system and nutritional needs.

OK read on to find out more about the Paleo Diet and some of the recipes you can try out.

Paleo Diet & Recipes

The recipes in this section take their inspiration from the currently fashionable Paleo diet. The recipes—

- have no grain products
- are low in carbohydrates
- contain plenty of protein
- contain good fats

I have given an example of a beef, chicken and fish meal as well as a simple dessert and salad.

The Paleo diet is based on the idea that for optimal health, modern humans should go back to eating whole unprocessed foods that are healthier for us. Over the past 200,000 years humans have adapted to whole foods: Plants, meat, seafood—all of them fulled with the nutrients our bodies evolved to thrive on.

Agriculture appeared on the scene only 10,000 years ago—a brief period of time in relation to man's appearance. There simply hasn't been enough time for evolution to completely adapt humans to eating modern foods like wheat, sugar, chemically processed vegetable and seed oils, and other processed foods. Many modern diseases—including immune disorders, cardiovascular disease, type 2 diabetes, and obesity have increased dramatically with the industrialization of food. The Paleo diet makes a health based case for a return to a more ancestral approach to eating.

Paleo-diet varieties

Some people won't eat potatoes or other starchy vegetables but you can easily create your own recipes by following these simple guidelines:

- Use wholesome forms of protein, organic if possible, such as beef or chicken
- Generally eliminate grain products like bread, cakes

and biscuits.

- Combine the protein with fresh vegetables, avoiding starchy types such as potatoes
- Avoid any grain-based product such as bread
- Avoid wheat based additives
- Use saturated fats such as pure butter, avocado and olive oil
- Use coconut oil for cooking
- Eat whole, unprocessed, nutrient-dense, nourishing foods
- Choose grass fed and pastured meats and eggs, wild-caught seafood, and vegetables.
- Add fruit, nuts, and seeds in moderation
- Avoid food grains, gluten based foods and sugar. These will produce inflammation in your body and lead to weight gain and bad health.

Many experts acknowledge the value of paleo-type dieting. I have personally come across a number of "hopeless cases" who turned their health around by following similar diets. Some paleo eaters choose to go low-carb, while others occasionally eat potatoes or a bowl of white rice.

Beef and vegetable stir fry

Ingredients

- 600g of sirloin or boneless beef
- two teaspoons five-spice powder or similar
- 3 tablespoons virgin coconut oil
- 1 small onion sliced
- 1 zucchini
- 1 and a half pounds julienne-cut orange and/or yellow carrots
- 4 cloves garlic, minced
- 1 teaspoon finely shredded orange peel
- 50ml fresh orange juice
- 50ml vegetable stock
- 50ml white wine vinegar
- One-quarter teaspoon crushed dried chili
- 6 cups cabbage sliced
- half a cup roasted cashews unsalted

Directions

1. Cut beef into very thin slices. In a bowl, toss beef and

five-spice powder. In a large wok, heat 1 tablespoon of the coconut oil over medium heat. Add half the beef; cook and stir for 5 minutes or till browned. Transfer beef to a bowl. Repeat with the remaining beef and another 1 tablespoon oil. Transfer beef to the bowl with the other cooked beef.

2. In the same wok, add the remaining 1 tablespoon oil. Add onion; cook and stir for 3 minutes. Add zucchini and carrots; cook and stir for 2 to 3 minutes or until vegetables are crisp-tender. Add garlic; cook and stir for 1 minute more

3. For sauce, in a small bowl combine orange peel, orange juice, Beef stock, vinegar, and chili. Add sauce and all the beef with juices in bowl to vegetables in wok. Cook and stir for 1 to 2 minutes or until heated through. Transfer beef vegetables to a large bowl. Cover to keep warm.

4. Cook the sauce, uncovered, over medium heat for 2 minutes. Add cabbage; cook and stir for 1 to 2 minutes or until cabbage is just wilted. Divide cabbage and any cooking juices among four serving plates. Top evenly with beef mixture. Sprinkle with nuts.

Chilli Chicken, Thai style with roasted peppers (Serves 4)

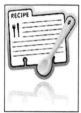

Thai-style roasted chicken legs are tender with just the right amount of spice and bite. They're great with roasted peppers, and easy to prepare. This is a simple recipe, bursting with flavor.

Use legs if you're on a tight budget: they're usually cheaper than breasts. Keep the chicken bones. They can be used to make chicken stock. Tapioca flour, used to thicken the sauce, can be readily found in health food stores. That keeps all the flavor on your chicken, instead of letting it run off into the roasting pan. Tapioca flour, unlike plain flour, comes from a root and not from grain.

This recipe offers a tasty alternative to ordinary chicken dishes and is a good way of using up legs.

Ingredients

- 4 chicken legs;
- 5 tbsp. white vinegar
- 50ml water
- 2 garlic cloves, minced;
- 1 tsp. fresh ginger, minced;
- 4 tbsp. liquid honey
- 2 tsp. pepper

- 1/4 tsp. cayenne pepper;
- ½ tbsp. rice flour;
- salt and fresh ground black pepper

Ingredients for the roasted peppers

- 4 bell peppers, halved
- 2 tbsp. virgin olive oil
- 2 garlic cloves, thinly sliced;
- 1/4 tsp. dried oregano;
- Sea salt and ground black pepper to taste.

Preparation

1. Preheat your oven to 400 F.
2. Season the chicken legs with sea salt and black pepper.
3. In a saucepan placed over medium-high heat, bring the white wine vinegar, water, garlic, ginger, honey, red pepper flakes, and cayenne to the boil.
4. Simmer and cook until reduced.
5. In a small bowl, combine the tapioca flour with 1 tbsp. of water.
6. Slowly whisk the tapioca mixture into the sauce and cook while stirring for a minute or two
7. Paint the chicken with the half of the sauce and place in the oven for 30 minutes.
8. Coat with the remaining sauce and roast for another 15 minutes.
9. Place the peppers, cut side up, on a baking sheet.
10. Drip olive oil over the peppers. Sprinkle with garlic,

oregano, and season with salt and pepper.

11.Roast in the oven until tender, about 30 minutes.

Fresh fish with herb sauce (Serves 4)
15 minutes prep and 15 minutes to cook

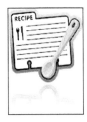

Use cod, snapper or gurnard for this recipe. The herb butter and coconut sauce give a creamy texture—a great alternative for those who find spicy recipes unappealing. The herb butter provides the cooking fat for the fish, but it also flavours the sauce while the fillets are in the oven. Don't throw out that browned butter in the pan. Use it on your plate.

Serve with steamed asparagus, garlic green beans, or new potatoes. A fresh salad or coleslaw makes a great side dish.

Ingredients

- 4 Fish filets
- 1 tbsp. chives, minced
- 1 tbsp. fresh parsley, minced
- 1 tbsp. fresh thyme
- 2 garlic cloves, minced
- 1 shallot, minced
- half lemon zest
- ¾ cup of coconut milk
- 6 tbsp. melted butter
- Sea salt and black pepper

Preparation

1. Preheat your oven to 400 F
2. Season each filet with sea salt and black pepper
3. In bowl, combine the butter, garlic, shallot, and herbs
4. Preheat a skillet over a medium-high heat
5. Pour the herb butter over the skillet and sear the fish on both sides
6. Place the fish in a baking sheet and cook in the oven for 7 minutes. Don't discard the skillet.
7. Pour the coconut milk and the lemon zest in the skillet that was used to sear the fish and bring to a simmer
8. Serve the fish with the sauce and lemon or lime wedges on the side.

Avocado Wrapped in Bacon Recipe
Serves 4 Prep: 10 min, Cook: 15 min.

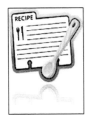

Avocados are usually eaten uncooked. If they are part of a hot recipe, they're sliced over a soup or taco, adding an interesting temperature contrast to the dish. But you can cook them. Wrapped in <u>crispy slices of bacon</u> and sprinkled with chilli powder, these mouthwatering snacks are sure to convert even the most stalwart avocado doubters!

Alter the amount of bacon on the avocado to match your taste. This recipe is easily prepared and provide a great snack while watching your favourite TV sport. The recipe is also suitable as an entree or side as an accompaniment to a main meal.

Ingredients

- 6 strips of bacon
- 1 avocado
- Chilli powder

Preparation

1. Preheat oven to 425 F
2. Line an oven dish with foil or baking paper
3. Cut the avocado into slices lengthways
4. Wrap each avocado slice with bacon. Sprinkle some chilli powder over the bacon-wrapped slices, and line them up on the baking paper.

5.Bake for 12 to 15 minutes

Banana Ice Cream
Serves 2/3, Prep: 15 minutes (6 to 8 hours to set)

All you need to make banana ice cream is bananas and a food processor. The results will surprise you. Sounds unbelievable. It's all due to the ability of bananas to stay creamy when frozen instead of developing hard crystals like most other fruits.

Normal ice cream is made from dairy, sugar and egg yolks vigorously churned by machine or by hand while the mixture freezes. Banana ice cream is easy to make and although not true Ice cream it's a great alternative.

This is an easy recipe to whip into to a creamy mixture. Adding extra ingredients such as cocoa, vanilla, fresh mint, chocolate or a few pieces of fruit at the mixing stage, gives you the possibility of endless flavour options for this great dessert.

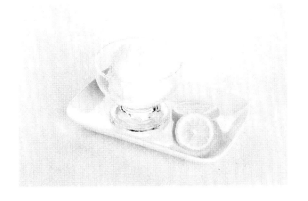

Ingredients

- 3 ripe bananas;
- Garnish with fresh fruit cut into pieces, coconut flakes, chocolate chips or flakes, chopped nuts or any anything else that grabs your fancy.

Preparation

1. Peel the bananas and slice into pieces
2. Place the pieces in a glass bowl and into the freezer overnight
3. Place the frozen banana pieces in the bowl of a food processor and mix until smooth. Scrap the sides of the bowl with a spatula as you go. It will take a while to become creamy.
4. The bananas will first become lumpy, then a very soft and creamy mixture
5. Place back in the glass bowl and in the freezer for a while to harden or enjoy it right away if you like very soft ice cream
6. Garnish with your favorite toppings and serve

Zucchini and Pine Salad

Ingredients

- Olive oil to coat
- 50g pine nuts
- 75ml virgin olive oil
- 2 teaspoonful lemon juice
- 1 teaspoonful liquid honey
- 150g mixed salad leaves
- ½ cup mint

Directions

1. Preheat the grill on high. Paint the zucchini with olive oil and season with salt and pepper. Cook for 3 minutes each side or until tender. Transfer to a bowl to cool.

2. Cook the pine nuts in a pan over medium heat, shaking the pan often, for a few minutes or until toasted. Place into a mortar. Gently pound with a pestle until crushed.

3. Place the crushed pine nuts in a small bowl. Add the oil, lemon juice and honey, and combine. Season with salt and pepper

4. Cut the zucchini into thick strips. Place in a large serving bowl. Add the salad leaves and mint, and

drizzle over the dressing. Toss to combine and serve.

Try these recipes or choose from thousands of others on the Internet. I'm sure you'll find plenty to suit your tastes. I'm going to give you 25 great weight loss tips in the next section.

9. 25 Weight loss tips

I had high hopes that I would benefit from these. My last monthly shopping trolley (six trolleys actually) contained a quarter of a million calories. And when I totted up all the chocolate bars, crisps and sweets I used to eat on my cycle rides in the old days I realized that my bike was in fact a mobile tuck shop.

There are some great weight loss tips in the following section, have a look but don't make the mistake I made playing games with the Wii. This was a bit of a disaster actually. I forgot to loop the handle round my wrist to avoid the controller flying off across the room. Managed to smash a vase and a Velux window and almost took the mailman's eye out.

1. Don't overdo carbohydrates. Most people new to cycling think they have to consume energy bars and drinks to keep up energy levels. The truth is unless you are cycling for more than two hours with reasonable intensity you don't need extra carbs, they will only end up as fat.

2. Eliminate wheat products. This is a biggie. Many top athletes find that eliminating or cutting down on bread, pasta and other wheat products and eating more rice, fruit and vegetables results in a leaner body.

3. If you have a food product you find hard to resist, remove it from your cupboard

4. Snack on nuts, seeds or dried fruit instead of muesli bars and biscuits

5. If consuming energy bars choose 100 to 200 calorie products or cut the bar into smaller portions. Most of these bars contain too many calories. They are good for athletes but not for regular exercise.

6. Try to eliminate processed foods. These contain sugars

which can cause an insulin spike. This disrupts production of the hormone that controls hunger. You are in an unhealthy cycle—the craving for sugar leads to the lay down of fat which in turn lead to renewed sugar cravings. The hormone that converts fat back to energy is disrupted, so you continually seek more carbohydrates.

7. Eat more fresh fruit and vegetables

8. Have a decent breakfast. A good breakfast means you are less likely to overeat snacks before your next meal. Eggs are ideal. Packaged cereals are full of sugar. If you tend to binge on food, eat small snacks during the day.

9. Explore your emotional triggers for overeating. If it's when you're unhappy try substituting a fun activity.

10. Monitor your food intake. Use a food diary or app such as "Lose It" to track calories.

11. Eat smaller meal portions. Buy smaller dinner plates. Stop eating when you're satisfied.

12. If you slip up one day and over-consume, don't beat yourself up, just start afresh the next day.

13. Eliminate soft drinks, they contain huge amounts of sugar. Drink plenty of water.

14. If consuming alcohol mixed with soft drink, eliminate the soft drink and use ice water.

15. Cut down on cheese

16. Weigh yourself weekly at the same time. People who regularly monitor their weight are better at controlling it.

17. Watching TV isn't good for your weight loss. There is a direct correlation between hours of TV watched and obesity. Try an activity like riding an exercise bike while watching TV.

18. Ride with friends and plan rides in your diary, you will

be more likely to keep up regular activity.

19. Stand, if you can, instead of sitting. Walk or ride instead of taking the car.

20. Take the stairs instead of the elevator.

21. Play real games instead of video games or use something like WIFit

22. Don't stay seated for longer than 30 minutes if possible without standing and walking around

23. Try to include your partner on your journey. It's been shown that people are more successful at losing weight and keeping it off if their partner is on the same wavelength.

24. Drink tea. Research suggests that those who drink tea—black, green, or white, have lower BMIs and less body fat than those who don't.

Now that you've read these tips pick out two or three to get started on. Commit to making them part of your routine. After a week or so add a couple more. Before long you will have made a lot of positive changes.

It's common for those who lose weight to complain that they can't keep the weight off. I will show you next how to keep that weight off for good and not stack it back on a few weeks later.

10. How to lose weight and keep it off

You've cycled regularly. You've watched the weight slowly fall away. You rejoice every time you look at your reflection in the window. Gone is the spare tire. In its place a svelte new you. Youth regained or at least a few years. Toned muscles have given your body the great shape you thought would never come back.

However, you need to be on your guard!

You can't take weight loss for granted. **At least a third of people who lose large amounts of weight will gain it back.** Your body has a built-in mechanism that aims to restore your weight back to its original level. Hormone induced hunger signal you to eat more food.

The good news is that if you exercise regularly every day you are more likely to keep the weight off. Sixty minutes of moderate cycling or 40 minutes of vigorous exercise is all you need.

Regular exercise, cycling included, burns more calories and helps control the hormone that produces hunger, effectively decreasing appetite. Exercise reduces the level of the stress hormone cortisol. This makes you more relaxed and less likely to eat for comfort.

Weight loss plateaus at a certain point. Further weight loss is possible only by exercising harder or by reducing calorie intake. Cyclists sometimes overeat in the misguided belief that the extra exercise means they need an increased food intake. By cutting your portion sizes you will help keep your weight down.

A significant number of people who lose weight and keep it off regularly weigh themselves. Weekly weigh-ins at the same time each week will enable you to keep track of your weight. And you can react to any slight gain by adjusting your food intake or engaging in a few harder sessions.

Set goals. When you meet them, set more. When I enter a race that is my goal for the weeks or months leading up to it. Once completed I target another suitable event sometime in the future so I always have a target to keep my enthusiasm up. You will find as your ability to cycle increases you will be able to achieve faster times and cover longer distances. This is great for your confidence and will help you keep up the enthusiasm to continue cycling.

Weight Maintenance

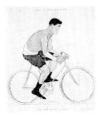

Up to this point I was losing weight. Then I read about unconscious mechanisms in the brain that throw a hissy fit if you don't immediately start munching your way back to the weight you were, in as short a time as possible. Why wasn't my brain speaking to me about this directly? What's with all the sneaking around? Was this Chuffer's doing?

My brain wasn't on my side. Great. If this was true then whose side was it on? There's a suggestion on how to thwart your brain's mutinous behavior and that is—wait for it—to exercise even more. Who would have thought it?

It gets worse. Seems like weight loss reaches a plateau. To continue dropping weight you either need to chop off a limb or exercise harder. Of course, you could also cut down your portion size. I sent away for a special plate. It was divided into sections—one for carbs, one for vegetables and one for protein. I could not believe how small the sections were. To get more than three potatoes on this plate you'd need to stack them one on top of the other. But then that wouldn't be cooking it'd be juggling.

I had previously tried several popular diets, which I adapted to my own needs. I invented the Atkins Plus. This entailed eating as much saturated fat as you could get your gnashers around plus anything else that took your fancy, any time you fancied it. I put on four stone in three months.

Setting personal goals is said to increase your chances of keeping weight off.

I set myself three goals:

> 1. I will enter a race at some point in the future
>
> 2. I will not eat so many pizzas (honest I won't)
>
> 3. I will try to be more active

Hmmm. These looked sooo lame on paper. Semantically, 'sometime in the future' included any time before I died. The 'eat less pizzas' goal technically included eating one less than normal. I was already ordering six trash can lid sized New Orleans Cajun Sizzlers a week so one less would make little difference. And as for trying to be more active, I could try to get into astronaut training but that was not so much a moon shot as a long shot.

Under the sheer weight of positive evidence on diet this book contained I immediately embarking on my 246th diet of the decade. I felt good about this. My train, I felt, was bound for Glory—well, maybe the station before Glory.

The next chapter promises to turbo-charge your weight loss so hold onto your hat and take a look.

11. How to turbocharge weight loss

Bike riding is a great way to lose weight and keep it off. I'm enthusiastic about it because I've seen it work for countless people. Getting in the cycling habit shifts the direct focus off weight onto the fun your having riding your bike.

Some people want to get rid of excess weight as fast as they can. This is not the healthiest choice. It *can* result in rapid weight loss but this is often followed by rapid weight gain. However, concentrating on a few aspects of your diet can turbo boost weight loss. As long as you don't go overboard you will lose weight fast.

I know you've heard this before but it's worth saying again: cut out the carbs. Carbohydrates not used for energy end up as fat. Most of us overestimate the daily amount of carbohydrates we need. Or else give it no thought at all. By cutting out or severely limiting the amount of carbohydrate in your diet and increasing the amount of good fats such as coconut oil, butter and olive oil your body will become more efficient at metabolizing fat. Diets such as the paleo diet are based on this fact.

Try this: for three days a week cut out as many carbohydrates as you can. Include bread, cakes, potatoes, pasta, and rice. What is left to eat you may think. Meat chicken, fish, nuts and soy are all types of protein that can be used to make great meals. Combine these with non-starchy vegetables.

For breakfast you could make an omelet with mushrooms, tomato, zucchini or any other non-starchy vegetable as a filler. For lunch make a chicken or tuna salad. For dinner try beef with stir fried vegetables.

Cook books are full of recipes that don't include carbohydrates. I included a few examples in a previous chapter. Use your imagination. As a bonus you can give yourself a decent portion size without worrying about it ending up as belly fat.

You could eat like this every day but many find it impossible to totally restrict carbohydrates. If this applies to you, three days a week should be achievable. Once your body becomes accustomed to a restricted carbohydrate intake you will find it easier.

Some experts say this does not qualify as a balanced diet. That's their opinion but the so-called 'balanced' diet they recommend has resulted in a worldwide obesity epidemic.

Try restricting cabs for a while. You'll be astounded how quickly you lose weight.

And you'll feel better for it too.

Ok Bruiser I know your busting to make your point, let's hear it.

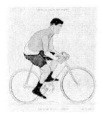

I am afraid I can't see the point of cycling to keep the mind off weight loss. I live in a perpetual state of hunger. In the same way that sharks must keep swimming or they die, I'd need to be in the saddle 24/7 or I'd have a litre of Ben and Jerry's down my neck before you could say 'Lance Armstrong'.

Nor did I go for turbo boosting by cutting out carbohydrates. Once you've binned carbs you'll have nothing to eat but the recipe book. Still, colour me stupid if I didn't try the no-carbs-until-Friday deal. By Saturday lunchtime I had already eaten my recipe book and I'd eaten a kilo of spaghetti before the six o'clock news. I'm cool with avoiding yo-yo dieting, though. Tried it once. Ate a yo-yo. Yuck.

I've just flicked through to the next chapter, "core exercises" sounds like peeling apples or something but let's read on.

12. Strengthen your body: Core Exercises

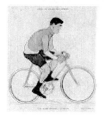

This section talks about 'sets' of exercises. You know the sort of thing—a bunch of geese is a gaggle and a bunch of cows is a herd. Well, a bunch of exercises is a set. The problem is they're all sets of ten or twenty. What's wrong with sets of one? Or none if you really think an exercise is going to hurt more than you'd like (that sort of exercise covers the vast majority)?

Just speaking the word 'exercise' out loud has always given me the galloping squitters. If God wanted us to exercise, he wouldn't have made it hurt when we performed a press up.

Most of the so-called exercises in this section are actually forms of torture (they are suspiciously similar to punishments handed out by the Spanish Inquisition). Some remain banned under the Geneva Convention. Consider The Plank for instance. This medieval abomination is supposed to exercise something called the 'transverse abdominal'. Wasn't Transverse Abdominal a Roman Emperor?

Then there's the delightful pastime of doing crunches on a Swiss ball. There's more chance of me doing squat thrusts on a Swiss cheese.

For those of us past our prime, doctors claim that any activity which causes you to get slightly breathless still counts as exercise. That's a boost for me, including as it does: Opening a tin of beans, licking a stamp, lifting or lowering the toilet seat, and winding up my alarm clock before bed.

Get serious now, no more putting it off, have a read all about core exercises and you'll be on the way to being a rippling cycling machine.

12. CORE EXERCISES TO STRENGTHEN YOUR BODY.

Good cycling requires strong core muscles. When your core muscles are strong, your body is more stable and able to deliver power to your legs. Incorporate these core exercises as part of your cycle training program. Start with two of the exercises then add more as you become fitter and stronger.

Plank

This exercise works the traverse abdominus, and the upper and lower back.

Lying flat on your stomach place elbows under your shoulders with forearms and elbows facing forward. Raise hips off the floor with feet raised on tip toes. Keep your back straight and tighten your abs. Hold for sixty seconds.

This exercise increases muscular endurance and muscle strength. This will help you while riding in the drops for extended periods.

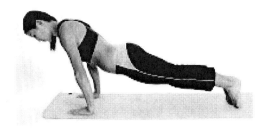

Crunch

This exercise works the traverse abdominus, obliques, and lower back. Lying face up with the middle of your back on a

Swiss ball, bend knees 90 degrees feet flat on floor, place hands behind neck but don't pull on your neck.

Squeeze abs towards your spine, keep shoulders off the ball and move torso in a clockwise oval motion. Press down on your lower back to keep the ball steady. Do ten clockwise ovals then ten anti-clockwise ovals. You have to move slowly and keep your abdominal muscles tight to keep yourself from moving around on the ball or rolling off.

This exercise builds stability in the core muscles and avoids wasted motion when riding on the bike.

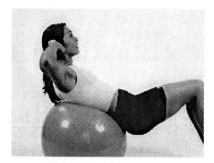

Traverse plank

This exercise works the traverse abdominus and obliques.

This exercise strengthens the obliques giving you better stability in the seat, resulting in better control and speed when cornering. Lie on left side with left elbow under your shoulder, forearm out for stability and lift your right foot onto your left, raise your right arm pointing length wise in front of you. Lift hips making a straight line down your side. Lower hips a few cm towards the floor than raise. Do twelve repetitions on each side.

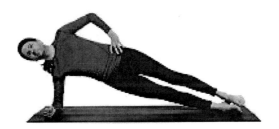

Bridge

This exercise works the lower back, glutes and hip flexors. Lying on your back bend knees with heels near your glutes, arms at your side, palms down. Squeeze your glutes, lift hips off the floor and push up with heels to form line shoulders to knees, toes off the floor slightly. Hold this for several seconds, lower halfway to floor (this is one repetition). Aim for fifteen to twenty reps. This exercise strengthens the lower back glute connection and stretches the hip flexors.

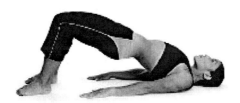

Boat pose

This exercise works the lower back and traverse abdominus. Sit with both hands behind, lean back until your torso is at 45 degrees. Keep legs together, lift them off the floor as you extend arms to shoulder height forming a 90 degree angle. This exercise builds lower back and core strength and stability and helps with your ability to stay bent in the drops for extended periods.

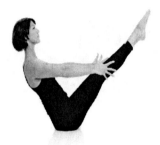

Swiss ball hip extension

This exercise works the glutes, lower back and hamstrings. Lie face down with hips and stomach on Swiss ball, hands under shoulders on floor, extend legs with toes on the floor. Keep shoulder blades back and lift both legs off the floor keeping them straight. Raise them slightly hold for several seconds and lower. Do fifteen to twenty repetitions.

These exercises are best performed in sets of three. The number of repetitions in each set depending on the individual's core muscle fitness level. Beginners should start with two or three reps per set and build up as your core muscle strength increases.

Start this week and do some of these exercises. Don't get carried away and overdo it. Otherwise you will suffer sore muscles over the next few days. Look for good form in the way you do the exercise rather than speed. You can increase the speed of the repetitions once you've got used to the proper positions.

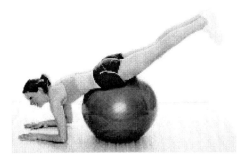

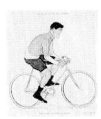

It didn't take me long to figure out how serious this chapter was. "Chuffers" first reaction was to try and convince me to flick past this and leave it until sometime in the future. 'No way,' I said. I used the motivational tips I learned to overcome my inner sloth.

I tried the crunches first (they're named after the sound my knees emit when I bend down. As for the "boat pose"—wasn't that the official stance when standing at the bow of an ocean liner reenacting a scene from Titanic. Anyhow, give it a go.

In the next section you'll find a program you can use to put your newfound poses into action.

13. Exercise program.

This program is a suggestion only. It's is a good idea to complete these after a cycle training session as your body is warmed up then. There's evidence to show they are more effective straight after a training session rather than completing them on a non-riding day.

Week 1 exercises

Three times weekly, preferably after a training ride

- 10 push-ups
- 10 crunches
- 10 bridges
- 15 second plank.

Week 2

Three times weekly after training (Do two sets)

- 10 push-ups
- 10 crunch
- 10 bridge
- 15 second plank.

Week 3

Three times weekly after training (Do three sets)

- 15 push-ups
- 20 crunch
- 15 bridge

- 20 second plank

Week 4

Three times weekly after training (Do three sets)

- 15 push-ups
- 20 crunch sit ups
- 15 bridge
- 20 seconds plank
- 10 boat pose

Week 5

Three times weekly after training (Do three sets)

- 15 push-ups
- 25 crunch
- 15 bridge
- 30 second plank
- 10 boat pose

Week 6

Three times weekly after training (Do three sets)

- 15 push-ups
- 30 crunch
- 15 bridge
- 30 second plank
- 15 boat pose

Next up is a program you can use for cycle training. It's a six week training program designed to help you lose weight. It's great for beginners as it starts out with a total cycling time of 20 minutes and builds up to 120 minutes at the end of the six weeks.

14.0 Six week "Bike to lose weight" programme

Use this plan as a guide. You can change the days or vary the times and intensities to suit, but try to follow the general idea.

On Monday you will ride for about 20 minutes. Start with a five minute warm up at low cadence and effort. Then ride for 30 seconds at 60% effort. After 30 seconds ride easy for one minute then repeat the cycle four more times. Then ride for five minutes at moderate pace with five minutes cool down at the end at easy pace.

When doing your hill intervals increase the cadence and resistance

Week 1	total	warm	
MON	20	5min	5x 30 sec at 60% effort, with 1 min easy between, then ride at moderate pace with 5 min at end to cool down
TUE	20	5	Ride this at moderate pace (conversational) for the ride cool down 5min
WED	40	5	Ride 5 min at 50% effort, then 5x 3mins at 60% with 2 min between.5min cool down.
THUR	20	5	20 minutes at moderate effort, easy spinning
FRI	20	5	Find some hills, do 3x 30 secs out of saddle with 90secs easy between.4 min easy spinning then 5 min cool down
SAT			Rest day
SUN	40	5	Sunday group ride at conversational pace.

Week 2	total	warm	
MON	30	10min	8x 30 sec at 60% effort, with 1 min easy between, then ride at moderate pace with 5 min at end to cool down
TUE	30	5	Ride this at moderate pace (conversational) for the ride cool down 5min
WED	45	5	Ride 5 min at 50% effort, then 5x 4mins at 60% with 2 min.between.5min cool down.
THUR	30	5	20 minutes at moderate effort, easy spinning 5min cool down
FRI	30	5	Find some hills ,do 5x 30 secs out of saddle with 90secs easy between.10 min easy spinning then 5 min cool down
SAT			Rest day
SUN	45	10	Sunday group ride at conversational pace.

Week 3	total	warm	
MON			Rest
TUE	30	5	Ride this at moderate pace (conversational)for the ride cool down 5min
WED	45	5	Ride 5 min at 50% effort, then 5x 4mins at 60% with 2 min between.5min cool down.
THUR	30	5	20 minutes at moderate effort, easy spinning 5min cool down
FRI	30	5	Ride 10minutes at 50% effort 10 min easy, then 5min cool down
SAT			Rest day
SUN	45	10	Sunday group ride at conversational pace.

Week 4	total	warm	
MON	35	5	8x 30 secs at 80%,1 minute between approx. 10mins moderate 5mins cool down
TUE	40	5	Ride this at moderate pace (conversational) for the ride cool down 5min
WED	50	5	Ride 5 min at 50% effort, then 6x 4mins at 60% with 1min.between.5min moderate, 5 min cool down.
THUR	40	5	30 minutes at moderate effort, easy spinning 5min cool down
FRI	35	5	5min moderate, hills 8x 30 sec out of saddle, 90 secs between spin easy to finish
SAT			Rest day
SUN	55	10	Sunday group ride at conversational pace.

Week 5	total	warm	
MON	40	5	8x 30 secs at 90%,1 minute between, approx. 13 min moderate 5mins cool down
TUE	50	5	Ride this at moderate pace (conversational)for the ride cool down 5min
WED	60	5	Ride 10 min at 50% effort, then 8x 4mins at 60% with 1min.between.5min, 5 min cool down.
THUR	45	5	35 minutes at moderate effort, easy spinning 5min cool down
FRI	40	5	5min moderate .Hills 5x 1 min , 90 sec between,15 min moderate, 5 min cool down
SAT			Rest day
SUN	90	10	Sunday group ride at conversational pace. Include 3x 30 sec intervals at fast pace with 90 sec easy

Week6	total	warm	
MON	60	5	10x 30 secs at 80%,1 minute between approx. 10mins moderate 5mins cool d
TUE	60	5	Ride this at moderate pace (conversational) for the ride cool down 5min
WED	80	5	Ride 10 min at 50% effort, then 8x 2mins at 60% with 1min.between.6min moderate, 5 min cool down.
THUR	50	5	20 minutes at moderate effort, easy spinning ,10 moderate pace,5min cool down
FRI	45	10	Hills 5x 2 min (alternate in and out of saddle)1 minute easy between
SAT			Rest day
SUN	120	10	Sunday group ride at conversational pace. Include 5x 30 sec fast intervals with 90 sec easy

Feel free to alter the programme to suit your individual requirements. As you progress, increase the intensity if you find you are doing the intervals without too much effort.

I know you're going to make excuses when it rains or you've run out of daylight to get out on your bike so in the next chapter we're going to look into how we can cycle indoors. You can just imagine what Bruiser's going to say about that!

15. INDOOR CYCLING

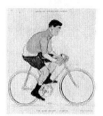

You learn something new every day. Apparently, when the weather's bad you can cycle indoors. Well I never. This is not encouraging. It is a long established routine of mine to sit down with a tin of Fosters in each hand to watch the late night weather forecast. I hope that any roads I plan to ride on the next day will be swept away by flash floods, cruelly condemning me to an extended bout of daytime television and popcorn binging. If cycling indoors was indeed possible then that small bit of excitement would be denied me.

But, if I was to give this cycling-back-to-fitness business a go, however half-hearted that go might be, I felt I might have to man up. Unfortunately I thought the means of transport for indoor cycling was the same road bike used for the highway. I leaped upon the Crimson Polecat like a seasoned rodeo-rider and started riding around the house randomly and at speed.

Though I was travelling much too fast to clock their facial expressions as I whizzed past them on the upstairs landing I was pretty sure my wife and children were unimpressed. Perhaps not as unimpressed as our insurance underwriters whose good offices covered us for accidental damage to home contents, but unimpressed enough.

By the time my wife stabbed a broom handle through the spokes of my rear wheel, bringing my rampage to an end by I had already trashed the den, dismantled our breakfast bar and driven headlong into my son's cello, turning it into matchwood.

Was I embarrassed when I discovered that the bikes used for indoor cycling don't actually go anywhere? Of course, but not as embarrassed as the first time I wore my Lycra cycling suit in public. Not by a long chalk.

Check it out for yourself, indoor training, not a bad idea if you want to hide your lycra clad frame from the public.

Indoor Training

It's hard to beat cycling outdoors and enjoying the environment. But sometimes it's not possible to get out on your bike. Bad weather will keep you indoors more often than you'd wish. And our busy lives often prevent you getting on your bike at a suitable time.

A regular cycling routine is an essential part of your weight loss programme. So what's to be done when you can't get to the Great Outdoors? Fortunately you can continue your training indoors.

Spin Bikes and Trainers

Spin bikes and trainers provide an effective means of continuing your training indoors. When you ride on one of these you are pedaling continuously. In doing so you will actually put in more work for the period than if you were riding outside where there are hills to coast down.

You are able to concentrate on effort without worrying about traffic and other distractions, hence put in a harder effort. These indoor trainers are ideal for interval training as conditions are the same for the whole session. If needed you can check your monitor or timing device without worrying about traffic or road conditions.

Spin bikes are stationery bikes which have a heavy flywheel. They are suitable for keeping in a single location because they are not easily moved, but you are able to do a great cycling workout on them.

There are several types of stationary bike—the upright stationary bike is perhaps the most common stationary bike. It resembles a street bike, but with gears in place of wheels. They don't require much space. They feel very natural, especially to the biker who really wishes to be out on the road. In addition, some upright bike exercisers claim that they obtain a better workout than riding on the street. That's because more effort is put into the ride on a stationary bike.

The recumbent stationary bike is another stationary bike option. It's great for people with balance or back problems. These bikes also offer more padding. In many cases, recumbent stationary bikes may be easier to ride and read or watch TV during the workout.

The dual-action stationary machine combines upright exercise with movable handlebars. This option gives the rider's arms a real workout. While many stationary bikes boast lower-body workouts, the dual-action bike offers better all-around total fitness. Usually these bikes are more expensive and larger than normal stationary bikes.

If you want to cycle, but age is a barrier, or you simply don't want to cycle outdoors, a stationary bike may be the answer. Workouts on stationary bikes are low-impact, yet enable the biker to burn lots of calories. Perhaps the best feature of a stationary bike is that the chances of coming to grief are fairly remote. No worrying about traffic and hidden potholes.

You can use your own bike indoors by attaching Turbo trainers to you rear wheel which rolls a drum. They are easier to transport so moving it in front of the TV is a great choice some nights. Turbo trainers come in different types and a range of prices. Generally the higher end products give the most realistic ride.

Indoor rides are best kept to short sessions as it is very boring and trends to be harder on feet and hands than out on a bike.

Here are a few points to make with regards to indoor training.

- Set up your indoor bike or trainer somewhere where

you can access it easily. If it is stacked away in a hard to get place you will be less likely to use it.

- If you can leave it setup ready to go that is ideal. Somewhere with a pleasant outlook or in front of the TV if you can. This will take the boredom off the exercise and you will be more inclined to use it on a regular basis.

- Regular exercise is an important part of a weight loss regime. An indoor setup will enable you to make up for those sessions outside you missed. It's also a great way for building your strength and fitness.

To keep your indoor training organized there's a one week programme next you can use to keep you heading in the right direction.

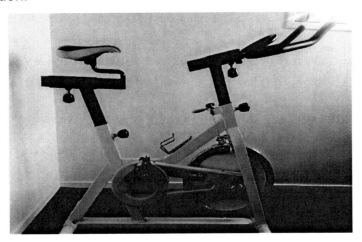

16. ONE WEEK SPIN PLAN FOR WEIGHT LOSS

You can repeat this programme each week increasing the resistance and intensity as you become fitter.

day	Time (min)	At the end of each session 5 minutes cool down, little resistance, no effort
Monday	30	10min warmup,10 x30 sec intervals at 50% effort.(1 min rest.between intervals at low resistance and effort) 5min at moderate effort
Tuesday	30	5min warmup 25 minutes easy at 40% effort moderate resistance
Wed	40	20 min moderate.3x 3min at 50% with (3 min at easy) between intervals
Thurs	30	5 min warm up.25 minutes easy effort ,moderate resistance
Friday	30	5 min warm up,5 minutes at 70% effort, moderate resistance,20 mins easy
Sat	rest	Go for a walk
Sun	50	5 min warm up, 3x3min at 80% effort moderate resistance.(1min easy low resistance between intervals) 33min moderate effort and resistance.

Establish the amount of resistance you need for moderate effort through some practice sessions. You want enough tension on the wheel so you can feel the pressure but not too much that it is hard to turn.

To explain Mondays session to you.

The total session should be about 30 minutes. First 10 minutes warm up at low resistance and low effort.

Do 10 intervals of 30 seconds at 50% effort and tension. Take 1 minute rest between intervals at low resistance and effort. Then take 5 minutes at moderate effort and tension. Finish off with 5minutes at low effort and tension.

After the first week you will get a feel to the amount of effort and tension you can put in. As the weeks progress, increase the effort you put in and tension on the wheel

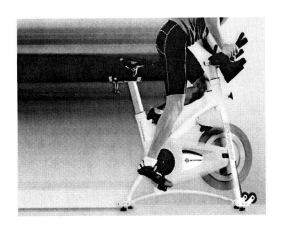

17. VACATION TIME.

Once you've become confident riding your bike you might consider including cycling as part of your next holiday. Cycling can offer a great alternative for your holiday or add an extra dimension to a regular itinerary. The great thing about cycling is that it includes physical activity. You will be able to cycle off those extra calories you may have overindulged on or just keep up your fitness levels. Cycling a scenic route adds another dimension to your sightseeing. You will experience far more of the surrounding countryside while cycling than you possibly could from a vehicle. Since the options are endless, cycling as become a popular activity to base your holiday on or add a highlight.

You can go on a cycling holiday virtually anywhere. Plan your own or use one of the many bike hire companies that offer guided or unguided tours. You can take your own bike or hire one at your destination. This type of holiday is appealing to individuals and families who want to experience the place they travel to up close. You can get to places that are inaccessible to vehicles. Streets, parks, mountains or virtually any place that appeals to you. If you are travelling with someone who isn't up to your fitness level, they could always hire an e-bike. They provide some motorized assistance, great for those hilly areas and a great way to include your partner who would normally struggle to keep up with you. Mountain bike trails are a great way to explore a new place. The popular ones are usually well marked and can add an exhilarating dimension to your holiday.

Cycling holidays have become popular. Many people base their holiday around the cycling. With the huge rise in popularity of cycling in recent times, the options being offered as part of an organized holiday are increasing all the time. If your budget is limited it's easy to organize your own routes and the only extra cost involved is transporting your bike or hiring one when you get to your destination.

If you've never considered a cycling holiday, give it some thought. You can visit some great places, explore areas that regular holiday makers will never see. You will feel that you really have experienced the area close up. The bonus is that you can stay fit in the process and not worry about your waistline increasing while enjoying the local cuisine.

Most people I know who have been on a cycling holiday or included a section of cycling, are so enthused by the experience they can't wait to start planning their next holiday. Give it a go I'm sure you won't regret the experience.

18.0 STAY ON TRACK

It's a good idea to keep a record of your rides. This is useful to be able to make a comparison over time to see how you have progressed. If you ride a regular circuit it will be easier to make comparisons with previous efforts.

You could use a simple diary to keep a record or purchase something suitable.

There are a number of different bike computers and speedos that monitor a variety of functions such as average speed, distance, calories used, elevation. It's up to you how much you want to record. For most recreational riders the distance, time and average speed are the most important functions. If you're watching your calories you might be interested in recording the calories consumed function.

If you own a smart phone you're able to use the free Strava App. I've found this a great way to record your ride.

Firstly it's free. At the start of your ride simply press the "record ride" function. At the end of the ride press the finish button. Within minutes a map of your ride is downloaded. All the statistics you need are recorded. You have an instant record of where you rode, the average speed, total time, elevation, calories consumed and more.

What I really love about this is the ability for you to make comparisons with your previous rides over the same course and with other riders who use Strava.

It is easy to mark a course or sections of a course for permanent record on Strava. Each time you ride the course or section, Strava will give you a comparison of your previous efforts. You will also be compared with any other Strava using rider who has ridden the same ride. This is gives you a great incentive to better your efforts.

When you are riding with a group of riders you can compare

your performance with their own over sections of the ride. I found it provided a great way to increase your motivation to bettering your performance. If you are out riding on your own you're are able to race the clock over sections of the ride or the whole ride and analyze your performance when you've finished. A bonus for those of you who are counting calories. You get a record of the calories you've burned up on the ride!

Ok Bruiser I know you're busting to say something.

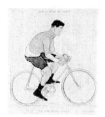

Keeping a record of my ride! That's the last thing I wanted to do at first. Imagine reliving the agony of those hills from the comfort of my couch and getting excited about it. No, I would rather watch the latest soap on the tele when I've finished riding my socks off. Well that's what I used to think. I have to admit once I'd got into this cycling for weight loss thing I started to notice a few things. The old spare tyre around the middle was disappearing and I was finishing my ride with some breath left over. I was getting into shape. I even asked Barry if he would join me for a ride. There was one stretch when I gave it heaps and left him gasping for air. Now that's something I wanted a record of. Saved on my smart phone for eternity, my ranking on Strava, number 265, Barry 270.

I was walking past the butcher shop the other day. You know the one where I first noticed my expanding midriff. I stopped dead in my tracks. A cursory glance in the window and who was staring back but Bruiser "mark two". I was looking back in time. My chiseled physique of way back was staring back at me. Well, call my dog a dingo, but I was amazed. Even my calves looked like they were manufactured at the wood turners shop. I was bathed in a glow of self-satisfaction. I had beaten the odds and become a cyclist for real. All the sprout sandwiches and boat poses had paid off. "Bike to lose weight" was my saviour.

19. CONCLUSION

If you've reading these words you're probably serious about controlling your weight through cycling. That's great.

The first step is easy. Get a bike and start riding. You've already learned how to motivate yourself, to get out riding and to keep at it.

Obviously what you eat plays a major part in weight under control. If you followed the tips I suggested and considered changing or modifying your diet don't be surprised when the kilos fall away. Cut down on carbohydrates and sugar in your diet and eat plenty of unprocessed wholesome food.

Cycling is an activity that will help you maintain a healthy body and lifestyle and is a great way to lose weight because gradually, your focus shifts from losing weight to riding the bike and weight loss takes place as a result of the riding.

 Whether you simply cycle for fun or move on to take part in organized events, cycling can become an activity that exceeds your expectations and opens up a whole new world of enjoyment to you.

You don't need to do the core exercises or execute my cycling plans to start cycling and lose weight. They will however, help you become a better rider leading ultimately to greater enjoyment.

Instead of sitting around snacking you are out taking part in an activity that will enhance your health and wellbeing. Remember, it probably took a number of years for you to get out of shape. So look at yourself as work in progress. As long as you are moving in the right direction the benefits will become more apparent. The speed at which you lose weight and gain fitness will depend on you.

Remember that bad weather needn't sabotage your efforts. Get on a spin bike or purchase some training rollers for your bike and include some indoor sessions.

Don't forget that holiday to reward yourself for all the hard work. Take your bike with you or hire one to explore your destination.

Good luck.

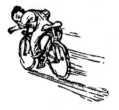

Bruce Fleming.

About the Author

I've been passionate about cycling and health and fitness for a number of years. I live in Sandspit New Zealand.

I am a qualified **Pharmacist** and also have training in **Nutrition** and **Natural Health** care.
I've been active in many sports over the years including surfing, Rugby, athletics, squash, hiking, martial arts and cycling.

Training and **Nutrition** are two of my great interest areas. For the last ten years **cycling** has taken first place in my sporting activities. I started cycling and found it a great way to keep fit and lose weight.
I follow training methods and nutrition trends and how these impact on performance..
I used to struggle to keep up with the bunch and was often totally wasted by the finish of the race and a long way behind where I wanted to finish. I'm now fitter and healthier than I've been for years thanks to the great benefits from cycling and some sensible eating. You can e-mail contactme@cycletrainingplans.com

Bruce Fleming.

RESOURCES.

Websites

- www.biketoloseweight.com tips for cycling and weight loss

- Cycle training for beginners tips on cycling, cycling plans, nutrition and other useful cycling information www.cycletrainingplans.com

CPSIA information can be obtained at www.ICGtesting.com
Printed in the USA
LVOW11s1702040116

468909LV00033B/299/P